Contributors

Billy Glisan holds a Master of Science degree in Exercise Physiology, and in his capacity with the Texas Back Institute, has worked in the areas of physical and motivational training for back patients. He has served as Director of Exercise Physiology, and as Director of Money Back, he developed an injury prevention program for the Institute.

Stephen Hochschuler, M.D., (consultant) is a board-certified orthopedic surgeon who specializes in spine surgery. He is a founder of the Texas Back Institute and a member of the American Academy of Orthopedic Surgeons. Dr. Hochschuler received his medical degree from Harvard Medical School and has recently been assistant clinical professor at University of Texas Southeastern Medical School.

The Texas Back Institute was founded in 1978 and serves thousands of back-pain sufferers who visit their Plano, Texas, facility in search of relief from mild to severely disabling problems. The Institute provides information and programs regarding muscular strength, flexibility, endurance, physical rehabilitation, therapy, first aid, injury prevention techniques, and general back problems.

Illustrator: Joanne Adams

Cover illustration: Marcy Gold

CONTENTS

CONTENTS

INTRODUCTION

Back pain and back injuries are very common in our society. In fact, approximately 60 to 90 percent of all U.S. citizens will experience at least one back injury in their lives. Half of these people will experience multiple episodes of back problems. Many will undergo surgical procedures, and roughly 10 percent will see their condition become chronic. The ultimate cost to society in lost productivity and health-care resources totals in the billions of dollars. An even higher price, however, is paid by the people who have lost the ability to participate in the activities they most enjoy. Back problems can make fishing, golfing, or even just playing with children and grandchildren fraught with pain. In the worst cases, a back problem can interfere with even the ability to get dressed.

Despite all this, people still take their backs for granted, not realizing the dangerous positions they put their backs in every day. Almost everything you do requires the use of your back, and back problems are rarely the result of a single activity or accident. Most injuries occur over a period of years or even decades, as a result of various factors—how you sleep or sit, what you eat, or how you deal with the emotional stresses at home and work.

But just because everyday life is filled with potential hazards for your back, don't think that you can never bend or lift anything again. On the contrary, your back is designed to move, bend, and twist. In fact, movement within certain ranges is healthy for the back. The key is learning the limits of these safe ranges and learning to live within them.

This book provides some low-cost, practical hints that will lower your risk of back injury and help you get through minor back pain. The combination of preventive measures and simple remedies will help your back stay healthy and pain free. However, this book cannot and should not take the place of a physician, therapist, or other health-care professional, nor can it teach you to treat serious back injuries.

The book is organized into six chapters. "Know Your Back" guides you through the various parts of the spine so that you can understand the relationships between the remedies and how the spine works. Next, "Immediate Pain Relief" describes some simple remedies for immediate relief of backaches or pain, including correct first-aid measures, the use of medications, exercises, massage, and finally, guidance on when backaches or pain are serious enough to warrant the attention of a physician. "Your Daily Routine" discusses the hazards of everyday activities and how best to prevent or reduce the negative effects on your back. "Exercises for Your Back" identifies and provides instructions for exercises that can keep your back strong and healthy. "Body Mechanics" focuses on correct lifting techniques and other proper body mechanics. Finally, "Other Lifestyle Factors" discusses the role of nutrition and stress in the life and care of your back.

Should you have any question regarding any of the information found in this book, feel free to call the Texas Back Institute's toll-free number, 1-800-233-0589, and talk to a HOTLINE nurse for free guidance on back pain or a back condition.

YOUR BACK BONES

In simple terms, your spine is nothing more than a group of bones in a line up the center of your back. The individual bones are called *vertebrae*. There are 33 bones in all— 24 vertebrae, the sacrum (which is actually 5 vertebrae fused together), and the tailbone, or coccyx (4 vertebrae fused together). The individual vertebrae are stacked on top of each other from about the level of your belly button up to your head.

When healthy, the bones of the spine are strong and dense. As is the case with all bones, the vertebrae get their strength primarily from two important minerals—calcium and phosphate. When there is a shortage or loss of these minerals because of an inactive lifestyle (weight-bearing activity actually helps to keep bones strong) or diseases such as osteoporosis, the bones lose their structure and strength. Unless they are weakened in this way or are damaged in an accident or fall, bones do not typically break or wear out.

The spine has four regions. Starting with the neck and progressing down to the pelvis, the regions are the cervical region, the thoracic region, the lumbar region, and the sacral region. All of these regions work together to provide support and stability for much of the weight of the upper body. Each bony level has a passage that forms a tunnel for the spinal cord, thus protecting the spinal cord as it extends downward from the brain.

But the spine is more than just a protective tube. While the spine provides protection and support, its design also allows you to bend, twist, rotate, and otherwise move your upper body in every direction. The bones themselves do not actually bend or twist; the flexibility of the spine comes from structures between the bones called *facet joints* and *intervertebral disks* (both discussed later in this chapter).

INTERVERTEBRAL DISKS

The infamous disks—technically known as *intervertebral disks*—are situated between the bones of the spine, creating a space for nerves branching out from the spinal cord to other areas of the body. The disks are made of tough rings of fibrous elastic material called cartilage; if you sliced a disk horizontally, it would look something like an onion cut through its middle. At the center of the rings of fibro-elastic tissue is a thick fluid with the consistency of very cold molasses.

Together, the rings and the jellylike center of the disk act as a shock absorber, much like the shock absorbers on a car. When healthy, they take up much of the shock that walking, running, jumping, and even sitting can place on your spine. Every time you bend, extend, or twist, there is a change of pressure in the fluid-filled area of the disk. In moderate amounts, this change of pressure is actually good for the disks. In the long term, however, excessive forward bending movements—with the back rounded and the legs straight—can damage the rings that hold the fluid in place. Unfortunately, this bending motion is one that many people use repeatedly throughout a typical day to reach or lift objects. Even slumped sitting may expose the disks to possible injury.

This damage to a disk starts at the rings in the center of the disk closest to the fluid, and then progresses toward the outermost rings. The condition has often been called a *slipped disk*. However, the disk does not actually slip out from between the bones. Rather, the fluid begins to break through the rings. When there are only a few rings left holding the fluid inside the disk, the condition is known as a *bulging disk*. The rings can push into the spinal cord or the nerves exiting the cord. If all the rings tear, the disk has ruptured, or herniated.

Some people experience a condition called *degenerative disk disease*. This condition usually progresses over many years. In this process, one or more disks dry out, losing their ability to absorb the loads and shock placed on them with everyday activities. Age also has an effect on the disks in the spine. At age 20, the disks are made up of about 70 percent water. With increasing age, the disks naturally lose their water content.

If a disk wears out, dries out, bulges, or tears, it loses height. This forces the bones closer together, so the facet joints end up having to take much more of the shock as you move. The facet joints, in turn, can wear out prematurely. The loss of height also narrows the opening between the bones through which nerves exit the spinal cord. This narrowing can pinch a nerve, often causing pain.

All of the conditions that affect the disk can, in the later stages, be extremely painful and debilitating. They can interrupt normal work, play, and even sexual function. Taking steps to protect the disks can pay great dividends in the long run.

LIGAMENTS

Attached to all the bones and disks in the spine are long, cordlike structures called *ligaments*. Not as hard as bone but not as soft as muscle, these bands of connective tissue come in almost every size. Some are short, running only between adjacent bones, but some are very long, extending all the way down the length of the spine.

The ligaments have several important functions. They provide support for the spine from the head down to the tip of the tailbone, holding disks and bones and muscles in their proper places. Their main function is to hold the bones together, allowing bending, twisting, and other movements to occur within safe ranges. Because ligaments are somewhat elastic, giving them the ability to stretch a little but not too much, they are perfectly suited for this task. When you bend over forward as far as you can, these ligaments reach the end of their length; they become taut, keeping the bones from moving apart any farther. This is an important function, because it spares other parts of the spine, such as the disks, the burden of holding the bones together—a damaging task that they are simply not designed to do.

The ligaments also play a major role in posture. When they maintain their normal length and flexibility, they support the bones of the spine, keeping them in good positions. With poor postural habits, however, the ligaments on one side of your spine can be overstretched. Over time, probably months or years, the result is poor posture. Poor posture, in turn, can cause the ligaments to ache. Indeed, back or neck pain that cannot be attributed to a specific accident or injury is often a sign that poor posture is taking a toll on the ligaments. The ligaments, when sprained or torn, take a long time to heal because of their poor blood supply.

MUSCLES

Muscles are cordlike structures that are even more elastic than ligaments. Like ligaments, muscles can stretch; but unlike the ligaments, muscles also have the ability to contract, or shorten. This is, in fact, what happens when you lift a cup of coffee, throw a ball, or do anything that requires movement of the body. The muscles shorten and lengthen, pulling the bones in different directions to coordinate our movements. When you lift, lower, push, pull, carry, or perform any activity, the muscles are doing the work.

Muscles also work to keep the body from moving when movement is not desired. For example, if you are sitting in a canoe and the canoe starts to tip to the left, your muscles quickly respond by coordinating your body's movement to the right to maintain your balance.

Muscles are true workhorses and can be your back's best friend. When conditioned, your muscles maintain their strength, endurance, and flexibility, which allows the body to move and work with less risk of injury and pain. When working properly, the muscles can greatly reduce the load on the bones, facet joints, disks, and ligaments. In contrast, when the muscles become deconditioned from lack of use or from injury, they tend to lose their size, strength, endurance, and flexibility.

How do muscles work? Basically, when you want to move, your brain sends a message through the nerves to the correct muscle. When the message gets to the muscle, chemicals inside the muscle cause the muscle to shorten. Because the muscle is attached to the bone, this shortening pulls on the bone. If the strength of this shortening is strong enough, the bone, and therefore the body, moves.

To lengthen, or relax, and return to its resting position, the muscle requires energy. If the muscle runs out of energy, or becomes fatigued, it cannot relax back to its original length. The end result may be what is often called *tightness*. As you use them, some of the smaller muscles in the back may start to get tired and shorten.

When the muscles shorten, the bones are held together more tightly than normal; this constriction, in itself, can cause back pain and limit your ability to move with full flexibility. In fact, many people have back pain that is probably related to tight, deconditioned muscles that have fatigued and shortened.

In the short term, this muscle fatigue may result in nothing more than a little low-level back pain, but if this condition continues day after day, year after year, the back can wear out much faster than it should. If the muscles are not stretched, they can be injured. If you're lucky, the injury will only be a pull or strain, in which the muscle is only slightly torn. Muscles can, unfortunately, be damaged more severely. The good news is that muscles, because of their good blood supply, tend to heal fairly quickly.

FACET JOINTS

Most of the bones of the spine have four joints, or places where they rub directly against other bones. These joints are called *facet joints*. Located on the extensions of bone off the back side of the vertebrae, these surfaces come in contact with those of the vertebrae directly above and below. Their purpose is to safely guide and restrict the movement of your spinal bones.

To get an idea of how the facet joints function, think of a door and doorstop. When a door opens so far that it hits against the stop, no further movement in that direction is allowed. In your spine, the bones move as far as the facet joints will allow them to before one bone forces another to stop. For example, when you stand and put your hands on your hips, bending as far backward as you can, it is the facet joints that help stop your backward movement. The same thing goes when you rotate your neck or back to the left or right as far as you can.

The surfaces of these joints, when healthy, are relatively thick, hard, and slick. This combination allows the bones an easy, pain-free gliding movement. However, if the joints are irritated, injured, or not used often enough in physical activity, the joint surfaces become thinner, softer, and almost sticky. This results in more difficult movement and possibly pain.

Without intervention, this condition can become chronic; bone spurs may even develop. Bone spurs are the bones' way of trying to grow together, or fuse, rather than remaining separate and moving freely. This condition can be extremely painful and may require surgery. However, it doesn't take such a serious condition to make these joints painful. If you've been standing on your feet too long, the facet joints end up getting compressed by the effects of gravity and the strain of supporting your upper-body weight, causing low-back pain even in healthy backs.

NERVES

Any discussion of the spine is not complete without talking about the body's messenger system—the nerves. In simple terms, the nervous system is similar to the electrical wiring in your home. The wiring system in your home carries electricity from room to room. The nerves carry electricity—in extremely small amounts—around to the different parts of the body.

The nerves actually begin in the brain, your body's command center, and branch out through the spinal cord, which runs through the bones in your spine. The spinal cord is the main information highway in your body; all of the brain's signals to the body are carried through the spinal cord. Where the nerves branch off and leave the spinal cord, they are called *nerve roots*. Beyond this point, they are simply known as nerves.

The brain is always monitoring what is happening throughout the body and sending messages—tiny amounts of electricity—through the nerves. The various parts of the body can, in turn, send signals back to the brain regarding their condition. The feedback to the brain includes important sensations such as pressure, heat, cold, movement, and the big one, pain. If damage occurs to the nerves, communication breaks down, and many problems can arise with the organs that require instructions or that need to report sensations.

Clearly, the spinal cord is vital to the functioning of your entire body. All of the sensations and all of the organs from your neck to your toes rely on that one telephone line. The other structures of the back (bones, muscles, and ligaments) can protect this pathway if they are properly maintained, but poor posture and bad habits can weaken your back's protective ability. Indeed, sometimes injury or strain to a muscle or disk can even affect the nerve root or cord itself, actually causing a nerve injury. And damaged nerves are not only bothersome—they hurt!

PUTTING IT ALL TOGETHER

All of these spinal structures and tissues work together to allow you to bend, move, or do essentially anything. It is a complex system with complex functions. Not only does your back have to support a good deal of your body's weight and carry vital nerve signals to all of the parts of the body, but you ask it to bend and twist at the same time. It is an engineering marvel.

Even though your back is very versatile, it does like certain positions better than others; that is, it can tolerate some postures or poses better. Specifically, the back is most comfortable while lying down with its natural curves aligned. In general, for sitting or standing, the more you can keep your curves properly aligned, the better it is for your total spine.

Moving, bending, and twisting in limited ranges is healthy for all parts of the back. Limit the forward bending of your back to about 30 degrees; this is a fairly safe range. A similar range exists for twisting of the back; you should try to minimize twisting motions to each side. Remember also that staying for extended periods of time in bent, twisted, or any awkward positions dramatically increases the physical stress placed on the spine. Certainly, the worst thing you can do to your back is combine all of these single factors by repeatedly bending over with straight legs and a rounded twisted back, then picking up something heavy at arm's reach, and then staying in this position for an extended period of time.

Your spine does benefit from movements that place acceptable levels of stress on them. Proper exercises can stretch, lubricate, and build the endurance of your back and strengthen its ability to withstand the forces of gravity in all of your movements. The most benefits are derived when these healthy movements are performed regularly. On the other hand, some people have problems with their backs because they have overdone it. They have performed the same movements too many times, and overuse has fatigued or injured certain spinal tissues.

1

REST YOUR BACK.

Even simple activities require some effort on your back's part. The activity need not be very demanding to cause a problem; maybe your back just isn't used to it. Often your back muscles simply overdo it. The end result may be a muscle pull or strain. In fact, most back pain and the majority of back injuries are probably related to muscle pulls and strains.

When strained, your muscles need a chance to turn off, rest, and begin to heal themselves. Find a comfortable position to allow your back to rest. The best position for an injured or achy back is lying down on either your back or side, with the curves of your spine in their natural position. Try lying down on a firm surface like a padded, carpeted floor. Place a couple of pillows under your knees. If on your side, place the pillows between the knees instead of under them. For your neck's comfort, roll up a small hand towel and place it under your neck to give it a break.

APPLY ICE TO REDUCE SWELLING.

Immediately after your back is injured, blood rushes into the damaged area. Even though swelling is part of the body's normal healing process, too much inflammation can increase pain and lengthen your recovery time. Applying ice immediately after a strain reduces the amount of inflammation, speeds up the healing process, and can numb some of the pain.

Generally, unless otherwise instructed by a physician, ice should be used instead of heat for the first 48 hours after a back strain. Heat from a hot shower, heating pad, or some popular topical lotion may feel better than using ice, but heat treatments increase blood flow, causing greater inflammation, more pain, and usually a slower recovery. At least for the first two days, stick with ice.

You do have to be careful with ice also, though. Incorrect application of ice can damage the skin. To apply ice correctly, warm a towel or pillowcase in slightly hot water, wring out the water, and quickly place an ice pack, ice cubes, or crushed ice in it. Immediately place the towel or pillowcase over the strained area of the back for *no longer* than 12 to 15 minutes.

If you do not have a towel or pillowcase handy, freeze water in a small paper cup. Peel the cup back so that the ice can go directly on the skin. Make sure that you continually move the ice around in circular motions, not allowing the ice to sit in one place. Another method is to place the ice in a plastic bag or some plastic wrap before applying it to the skin. For additional benefits, use repeated ice treatments approximately once every hour for the first 24 to 48 hours after the strain. This should help to keep swelling to a minimum and reduce the related pain.

COMPRESS THE AREA.

Gently compressing an injured area can assist ice in reducing inflammation and pain, while speeding recovery. Compressing the muscles can provide some temporary support for the area, which may allow you to move around more easily while making you more comfortable. Try using an elastic bandage; wrap it around your midsection over the strained area of the back. Make sure you do not wrap it too tightly. (The wrap can be used over an ice pack, provided the ice is applied as described in remedy 2 and for no more than 15 minutes.) An alternative to the elastic bandage is a back support, which acts like a corset to compress and support the back and stomach muscles.

4

TAKE ASPIRIN, ACETAMINOPHEN, OR IBUPROFEN.

Nonprescription drugs such as aspirin, acetaminophen, and ibuprofen have the ability to reduce back pain and, to some degree, inflammation. Some physicians, when prescribing medications for back pain, prefer aspirin or ibuprofen to treat pain that comes from muscles, ligaments, and bones.

The difference between over-the-counter and prescription forms of these medications is really the dosage, or amount, of the drug in each pill or tablet. Unless instructed otherwise from your physician, stay with the recommended dosage listed on the manufacturer's label. When you exceed the recommended dose, you increase your risk of experiencing the negative side effects of the medicine.

5

KNOW WHEN YOUR CONDITION REQUIRES A PHYSICIAN.

Muscle pulls and strains, although quite common, can be severe. Other spinal tissues can also experience injuries. Ligaments can be sprained or torn, and of course, spinal disks can bulge and tear. It is important for you to know when a back injury goes beyond your ability to treat yourself.

After a strain or injury to the back, the body can have a variety of natural reactions causing numerous symptoms, such as back pain. If, after two or three days of bed rest, your severe back pain has not subsided, you should see your physician. Sometimes, when many of the tissues in the back are seriously injured, the muscles can tighten up, or spasm, and clamp down around blood vessels. Muscle spasms can cause pain, sometimes severe, that makes it difficult to sit, stand, or do virtually anything. Many times, the only way to relax intense spasms is with the assistance of a physician.

Other signs to watch for are the loss of bowel or bladder control or pain, numbness, tingling, or other similar sensations that run down an arm or leg or around the chest. This type of symptom can make your hands, fingers, feet, and toes feel like they are burning, cold, asleep, or being poked with pins and needles. Finally, it's time to see your physician when it takes larger and larger amounts of medication to reduce your back pain.

If you experience any of these symptoms, get a professional opinion. Serious injuries that go untreated or are treated incorrectly can be dangerous, leading to further impairment and possibly irreparable damage. Just having one of these symptoms does not automatically mean that you will require major therapy. However, it's best to let your physician rule out serious spinal problems so that you can put your mind at ease and get on with the business of healing.

6

ALTERNATE HEAT OR ICE WITH STRETCHING.

As mentioned, muscles often spasm, or get tight, as the result of a back injury. This can be quite painful. Tight muscles and most sore joints do respond quite well to heat (topical lotion, hot shower or bath, heating pad), because the warmth relaxes tight muscles, increases blood flow, and eases pain.

Gently stretching these muscles after the heat application can further relax and lengthen tight tissues, easing movement and reducing pain. Remember, though, in an acute injury, don't use heat until after 48 hours, because it can increase the swelling and slow your recovery. In the first 48 hours after an injury, ice is the better alternative, and ice can also be used with stretching. Ice works a little bit differently than heat; it tends to numb the sensation of pain in sore muscles, which allows you to stretch and relax tight muscles gently.

The use of heat or ice is a matter of personal preference, and you have to experiment with each to determine which works best for your particular strain or injury. Try applying heat or ice as suggested for 10 to 15 minutes, and then see if performing the stretches helps your back pain subside. Be careful not to overstretch. Overstretching can aggravate a bad back, increasing pain and possibly causing re-injury. To stretch correctly, take a stretch only to a point of mild tension, not pain. Hold the stretch at this point for at least ten seconds, making sure that you do not bounce on the stretch. Relax the stretch and repeat right away two or three times.

Your muscles are kind of like springs. They tend to stretch fairly easily if you stretch correctly, but they tend to come back to their shortened position over the course of a few hours. So you will probably have to repeat these stretches throughout the day. Finally, if your pain or symptoms increase, stop the activity and consult with your physician or therapist.

7

AVOID HARMFUL ACTIVITIES.

The body starts its healing process as soon as an injury occurs. You can help this process by avoiding activities that might make your back condition worse. Depending on the degree of damage to your back, many activities you perform on a daily basis can be stressful to an already sore back. When your back is recovering from a strain or injury, you should consider avoiding or at least being extra careful with certain activities.

Avoid obviously stressful activities such as shoveling, in which the back is often twisted while lifting the weight of the shovel and its contents. Loading and unloading groceries from the back seat or the trunk of the car can quickly irritate your back even if the groceries don't weigh too much. In the same vein, be careful picking up children. It can be very easy to forget how heavy a small child is. Also, hoisting a toddler up to give him a hug is not usually considered strenuous work, so you may not realize the potential hazard it presents to your back.

You also must watch out for less strenuous activities that you might not associate with back stress and pain. Not every movement that is dangerous comes with an obvious warning sign. For example, chores such as raking or vacuuming can be very stressful to the spine, because reaching causes the spine to rotate, a motion that an injured spine may not be ready to do. Even doing the laundry, especially bending to remove heavy, wet clothing from the washer, or washing the dishes can wreak havoc on a painful back.

As your back starts to heal, gradually add these activities back into your daily life as your back can tolerate them, but remember, your back takes time to totally rebuild its strength and stamina after a strain or injury. Don't rush it.

PRACTICE GOOD POSTURE.

Couches and recliners can feel very comfortable; however, very few are designed with the health of your back in mind. If you are going to sit, try not to slump or slouch. Poor posture, such as slouched sitting, can place a great deal of stress on your muscles, ligaments, and disks. This stress can make it more difficult for proper healing to occur and may increase back pain. Choose postures and positions that allow you to keep the curves of your back aligned. Try rolling up a towel to about the size of your forearm and placing it in the small of your back to support the curve of your low back. If this feels uncomfortable, see if rolling it smaller helps. Remember to support your neck, as well.

TRY A MASSAGE.

Your muscles operate kind of like your car's engine. As they work, muscles accumulate waste products that need to be removed like the exhaust from your car's engine. If these waste products do not get out of the muscles promptly, then the muscles don't work very well. Furthermore, the buildup of these waste products can even create pain. A gentle massage helps to relax tight muscles, open blood vessels, and flush out these waste products, allowing the muscles to work normally while reducing pain and stiffness. Using an over-the-counter topical lotion that contains a heat agent such as mentholyptus can further increase blood flow and comfort by enhancing the relaxation of muscles and blood vessels; follow the package directions.

10

KEEP MOVING.

Even though rest is important for an injured back, too much rest can actually make your back worse. Let's say you have hurt your back, so you lie down on your back on the floor or couch or in bed for a week. Your decision to lie down may have been a good one in the short term—for a few hours or even a couple of days. The rest will allow your back to heal. In the long term, however, lack of movement robs the spine of its health.

After a couple of days of inactivity, even healthy muscles start to lose their strength and flexibility—they begin to atrophy. The longer you are immobile, the greater the loss. But muscles are not the only ones that suffer. Movement is vital to the other structures of the back, also. The intervertebral disks receive their blood supply from the bones above and below when you move. Inactive bones that are not bearing any weight become weaker and more brittle. So in essence, movement strengthens and feeds your spine, whereas inactivity weakens, starves, and decreases its life span.

Although your back may need short periods of rest in a sitting or lying position, you should try to change your position from lying to sitting or even walking if you can tolerate it. While you're lying down or sitting, try engaging in an activity that requires the gentle use of your hands and arms, such as knitting or some other handiwork. Whether you know it or not, using your arms, hands, or even your feet in this way is actually a low-level back exercise that will strengthen and feed your spine.

As your condition improves, increase the amount of time that you spend on your feet, performing light activities that require limited bending and twisting movements. Be especially careful with lifting and lowering activities. Gradually progress toward activities that include the bending, limited twisting, and light lifting that your back can tolerate.

GET A BACK-FRIENDLY BED.

Many activities in a typical day put stress on your back—even some activities that you may not think of as strenuous at all. In the short term, these activities may result in minor aches and pains; in the long term, they can cause chronic back problems. For example, about a third of your life is spent in bed. Still, some people never make the connection between their early morning back pain and the condition of their bedding or how they position themselves in bed at night.

When was the last time you bought a new bed? Maybe you considered putting a sheet of plywood under your mattress to support your back. Many sleep-related backaches are indeed caused by a mattress that is too soft. In most cases, however, adding plywood to a soft mattress will not help, because there is just too much soft material between the wood and your body, and your spine gets too little support.

What you need is something firm. Many people like lying on a carpeted floor, because it is firm but has some padding on top of it for your bones. This might work sometimes, but what you really need is a good orthopedically designed box spring and mattress. The cost may scare you at first, but consider how much money many people spend on car payments every month; think how much time the average person spends per day in that expensive car or truck; now consider how much time you spend in bed. Get the picture?

What kind of mattress is best? That may come down to personal preference. Different types of bedding, such as water beds and air mattresses, have different advantages and disadvantages when compared with more conventional beds. For example, a water bed, when filled with the proper amount of water, can have a therapeutic effect. The heat of the water may keep your back more limber as you sleep. On the other hand, if it has too much or too little water, your back may be stiff in the morning—if you manage to sleep that long.

Whatever your choice, gauge your bed's support by lying down on the bed in your usual sleep position (on your back or side—

not on your stomach), and have a friend look to see if your spine is aligned correctly. Imagine a line drawn through the ear, the shoulder, and the hip joints on one side of your body; if the line is straight, then the bed is OK for you. If you share a bed with someone, make sure that he or she is also lying in the bed before trying this out, because the change in weight will definitely make a difference.

Finally, what is the best position to sleep in? Sleeping on your back or side is usually better than sleeping on your stomach. The problem with lying on your stomach is the position that your neck and head are forced into. With the right mattress and pillows, most people can lie on their stomachs and everything will line up perfectly, but the neck ends up having to twist or rotate to one side because you can't breathe with your face straight into a pillow. The end result may very well be a stiff or sore neck in the morning.

12

STRETCH BEFORE GETTING UP.

As you sleep, your body shifts blood and warmth from the back muscles to the kidneys, liver, stomach, and other organs that need them all night. When you wake up in the morning, the lack of blood flow and movement in your spine makes it vulnerable to strains and sprains. Face it, your back is just not ready for the day.

To reduce the risk of back strain or injury, stretch before you get out of bed. Lying on your back in a relaxed, comfortable position with your legs extended, slowly raise your arms over your head and lay them on the bed. Gently reach with both arms as far over your head as you comfortably can. Then, add your legs and toes to the exercise, pointing your toes toward the foot of the bed. Remember to stretch only to the point of mild tension, hold the stretch for ten seconds, and then allow your whole body to relax. Repeat this stretch a few times. For your spine, it's like breakfast in bed.

13

USE THE LOGROLL TECHNIQUE TO GET OUT OF BED.

Getting out of bed may not seem like much of a problem for your back. If you have ever had a back injury, though, you probably found out that this seemingly easy task can be one of the most challenging feats you attempt all day. The first thing you can do is make the task easier by raising your bed off of the ground if it sits flat on the floor (the way many water beds do). If your bed is on the floor, put it on a pedestal or bed frame. It makes the task of getting out of bed much easier on your back and the rest of your body.

Next, use what is called a *logroll* to get your body in a position to get out of the bed. The technique goes like this: As you are lying on your back, roll over onto your side so you are facing the side of the bed you plan to get out of. Gently bring your knees toward your chest, keeping your legs in contact with the bed at all times. As you do this, simultaneously use your hands and arms to push your upper body up off of the bed; let your legs fall slowly off of the edge. As your upper body raises up, most of your weight will be on the hip, buttocks, and thighs rather than on the spine. Complete the maneuver by extending your back up as you push yourself up and out of the bed. Keep your back straight and your head up.

Take your time completing this maneuver. Remember that your back is still waking up, and even after an in-bed stretch, it is not entirely up to speed. A little extra time and a little extra care spent here could save you the agony and frustration of a bad back day.

Remember, getting back into bed can also be stressful to even a healthy back. It can be tempting to flop into bed at the end of the day, but the forced twisting that such a fall can cause is dangerous. So to ensure a safe and restful evening, use this technique in reverse to get back into bed.

1 Roll to face the side of the bed, and bring your knees up toward your chest. **2** Push your upper body off the bed while letting your legs drop off the side. **3** Keeping your back straight, rise off the bed with the aid of your arms and legs.

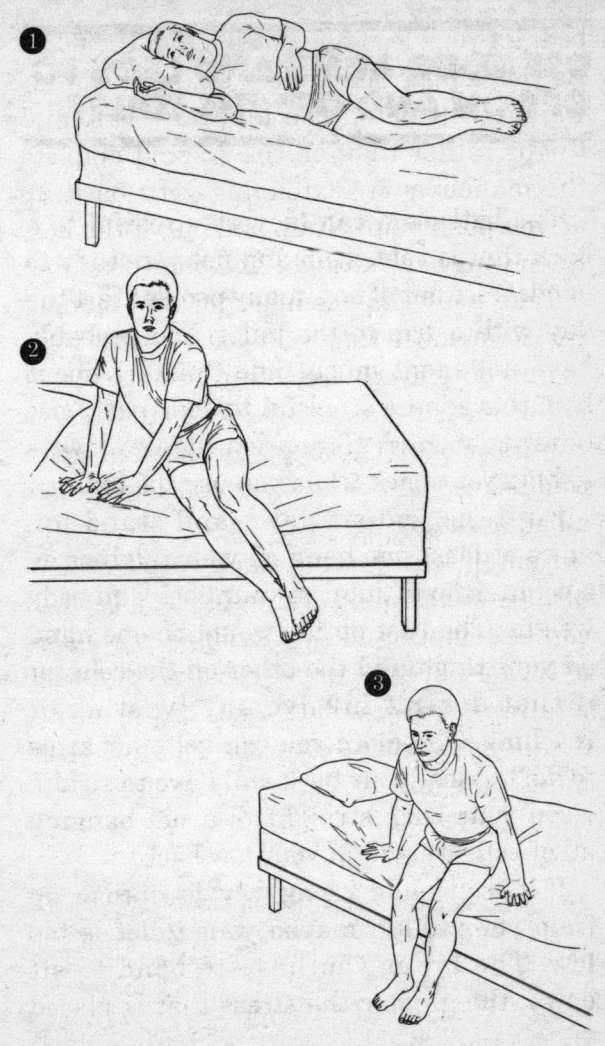

14

USE YOUR ARMS AND LEGS TO GET ON AND OFF THE TOILET.

The bathroom can be very stressful to a back that is cold, stiff, and not yet ready to bend. Once out of bed, many people start the day with a trip to the toilet. You probably have not spent much time thinking about how this can be stressful to your back, but hazards abound. Here are a couple of ways to help your back when you use the toilet.

First, as you sit down and stand up, place at least one hand on your thigh or on a countertop to support your back and body weight. The best option would be one hand on your thigh and the other on the counter if that doesn't involve any twisting or reaching. The more you can get your arms to do, the less your back will have to strain. Keep your back straight to avoid hanging all of your weight on your low back.

If it seems like a long way down to or up from your toilet, maybe your toilet is too low. The lower you have to bend to sit down, the greater the stress that is placed on the low back. An elevated seat cushion can be purchased from a medical supply store. Pay attention to where your toilet-paper holder is situated. Some toilet-paper holders are placed behind the toilet, forcing you to twist your back around to reach the paper. This movement is not good for a healthy back that is warmed up and stretched out, let alone for a cold, stiff back that just woke up. If the toilet paper is behind you, move it. Some people choose the toilet as a place to read the newspaper or their favorite magazine. Choose a friendlier location for your back.

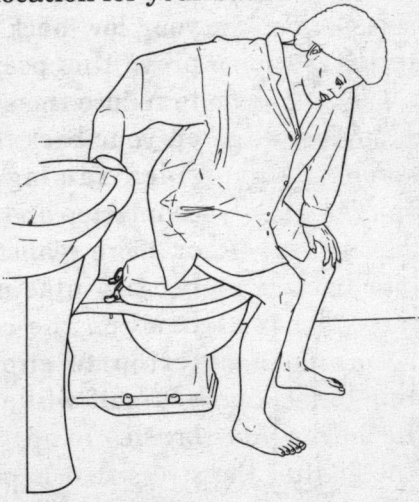

15

USE YOUR ARMS TO SUPPORT YOUR BACK.

Sinks can be the next challenge for your back. Sinks are built too low for many people. Brushing your teeth or washing your hands can place a lot of stress on your back. Next time you brush your teeth, stop and check what position your low back is in. Odds are that you will catch yourself standing bent over the sink with all of your upper body

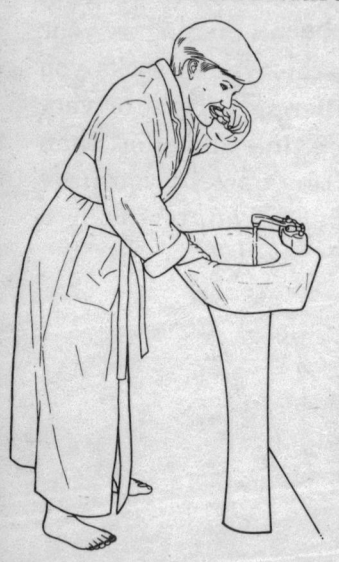

weight hanging on your low back. Improve this position to reduce the stress on your back. Consider raising the countertop and sink or, more realistically, try placing a hand on the countertop to support yourself while you brush.

16

LET YOUR FEET HELP YOUR BACK.

Forced bending and twisting of the spine is one of the worst activities for your back. Does sitting on the edge of the bed, with your feet on the floor and then bending over and twisting to put your socks on sound familiar? A way of making this task easier on your back is to bring your feet up toward your back. Try placing your heels on the edge of the bed or a chair and then putting on your socks or shoes. Also, the type of socks you wear does make a difference. Tight or very tall socks require more time and effort than do short or looser-fitting ones. If you have trouble getting your shoes on, try using a shoehorn.

17

GIVE BACKACHES THE BOOT.

Shoes play an important role in the comfort of your back. Flat, thin-soled shoes often increase your back discomfort. Look for shoes with good arch supports and a fair amount of soft material under the heel to absorb the shock created when you walk. If you cannot find a shoe that meets these requirements, look into silicone or rubber shoe inserts.

Women may experience low-back pain when wearing high-heeled shoes—and not without reason. As you remember, the low back should have a slight inward curve to it. High-heeled shoes greatly exaggerate this curve and can compress the facet joints of the spine. Wearing a lower heel is usually a better choice for your back. If you work in an environment that requires you to wear high-heeled shoes, wear a pair of athletic shoes to work and then change into your dress shoes at work. Men need to watch out for a similar problem if they wear boots with tall heels.

18

RIDE RIGHT.

If you are like most people, you probably use your car to go almost everywhere. Many people have to travel long distances to and from work each day. Most people do not take the time to adjust the seats in their cars, but a properly adjusted seat can reduce the stress and strain on your back. Try the following adjustments next time you use your vehicle.

Bring your seat close enough to the steering wheel to minimize the reach for your hands to grasp the wheel. Your legs should be bent at the knees and hips rather than kept straight. If you have an adjustable lumbar support, adjust it to where you have a slight inward curve in your low back. If your car does not have this feature, roll up a towel to about the size of your forearm, and place this in the small of your back. If your seat has a tilt adjustment, start with your body sitting up perfectly straight, and tilt it slightly backward but not too much. Keep your buttocks against the back of the seat so that they do not creep forward, causing you to slump.

If you travel long distances, or sit in the car for long periods, make slight but frequent adjustments in your seat's position. Even if your seat is adjusted perfectly and your back is aligned just right, locking your spine in one position for the length of the ride can cause you a lot of problems. Remember, your back likes movement. Those slight shifts keep it happy and healthy.

If your job requires you to be on the road constantly, you might want to make seat adjustability a priority in your next car purchase. In your present vehicle, though, there are various seat cushions and inserts that you can buy to improve your back position and to make your driving more comfortable. Let your back guide you in your purchase—one size does not fit all.

19

EASE IN AND OUT OF THE CAR GENTLY.

Besides the ride itself, your car presents other hazardous situations for your back. You may not pay too much attention to how you get in and out of your car. Some people almost fall into their cars, twisting their backs in potentially dangerous ways. Getting out can be equally strenuous and hazardous if you are not paying attention. Here are a couple of helpful hints to lessen the strain on your back as you get in and out of your car.

Before you get out of your car next time, move your seat back away from the steering wheel as far as it will go. Open the door all the way, and place your right hand on the steering wheel and your left hand on the edge of your seat, next to your left thigh, or on the edge of the roof. Lift both legs off of the floor boards, keeping them together, and move your legs and upper body as a single unit toward the open door. You should feel like you are spinning on

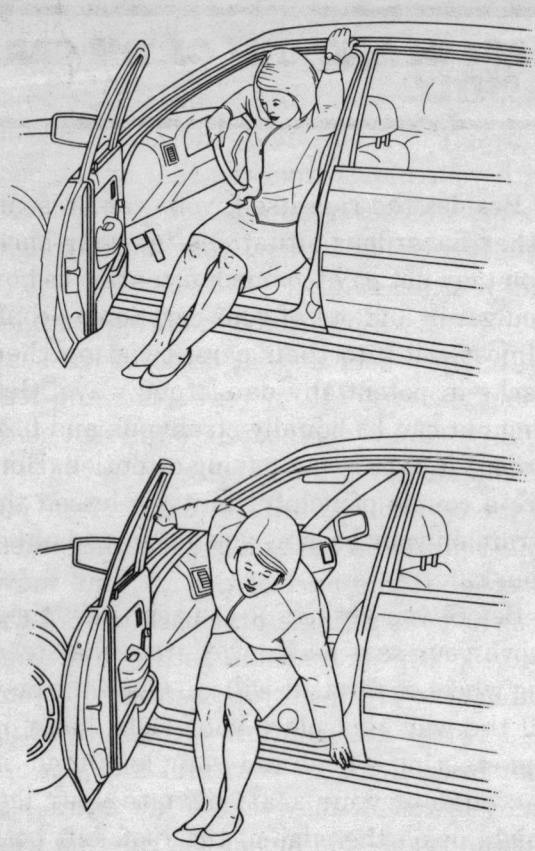

With a firm grip on the wheel and either the roof or the edge of your seat and using your arms to support the weight, spin your body to face the side *(top)*. Keeping your back straight and head up, stand up by pushing off from the door frame or seat *(bottom)*.

your bottom, without twisting your spine. Next, put your feet on the ground and use your legs, hands, and arms to help raise yourself up and out of the car. Push off with your hands from the seat or the door frame, whichever affords you better leverage. Remember to keep your back straight and your head up.

To get back into the car, turn your back to the open door and sit down in the seat, using the strength of your arms and legs again to lower your body into the seat slowly. You should still be facing off to the side of the car, not toward the front. Next, put your right hand back on the steering wheel or other stable part of the car, and move your body as a single unit back toward the steering wheel. Just like getting out, your whole body pivots on your bottom and your legs swing into position without twisting your back. Readjust your seat and you are ready to roll. It may take a few extra seconds to get in and out of the car this way, but in the long run, it will help keep your back free from aches and pains.

20

FEED YOUR SPINE.

Even with a perfectly adjusted seat, the lack of movement that goes along with a car ride starves your spine. On long trips, get out of your car as frequently as possible. When you make a stop, stand up, place your hands on your hips, and gently arch your back. This will relax and stretch tight, tired muscles and help to keep the joints lubricated. Like all stretches, remember to hold the position for at least ten seconds.

In addition to stretching your back, you should stretch your legs. Stretching your legs directly affects your back and can easily be accomplished with a short walk or by putting one leg on the bumper of your car and slowly straightening your knee until you feel a mild stretch in the muscles in the back of your thighs.

21

LET YOUR BACK REST AT WORK.

Office work usually requires a great deal of sitting, which can increase the stress placed on the back. However, you can improve your back's tolerance to sitting in the office. Start with a good ergonomically designed chair—a chair designed to fit and support the body and spine. Ergonomically designed chairs can be expensive, but in the long run, not as expensive as a damaged back. Whether you have the most advanced ergonomically designed chair or if you have to live with what you have, try the following suggestions to fit your chair to your spine.

Start by sitting all the way back in your chair so that your buttocks are up against the bottom of the back rest. Let your back lean against it so that the muscles can turn off. You may have been trained to type sitting up in a chair without leaning back against a support. This might be good posture, but it's very tiring for your back muscles. A footrest that lifts your knees to about the height of your hip joints will help you maintain the proper position. If your thighs are too short for the seat pan (the part you sit on), buy a cushion that will act like a spacer between you and the back of the chair. You should be able to sit all the way back yet still have some space between the backs of your knees and the seat pan.

Adjust the lumbar support to fit your low back's natural inward curve. Also, make sure that the lumbar support is set in the right place—about the height of your belly button. If you do not have a lumbar support, add one by using a rolled up towel.

Many aches and pains in the upper back, and possibly even headaches, may result from the muscles of the upper back growing tired of supporting the weight of the arms. Armrests support the weight of your arms and allow your neck and shoulder muscles to relax. Some people use a wrist rest to support the weight of their arms when they do not have armrests on their chairs. These can certainly help, but be careful to use them correctly. They are designed to support your wrists and arms when you stop typing, not while you type.

22

SET UP YOUR WORKSTATION CORRECTLY.

How you treat your back at work is very important, but how you organize your office equipment is also important. These days, very few jobs do not involve a computer, and many computers are set up very poorly. Incorrect placement of your computer can cause neck, shoulder, and back pain and even headaches. Check the following to ensure that your computer equipment is placed correctly. First, as you face your desk or workstation, make sure that your monitor and keyboard are set directly in front of your chest so that you do not have to turn your head to the side or twist your back. Second, ensure that the monitor is set at the correct height. For most people, this means that you should set the top of the screen at eye level. (Be sure that you have adjusted your chair and are using good posture before you make this determination.) Third, if you type a lot from paper documents, get a document holder that attaches to the side of your monitor.

If the majority of your computer usage involves text entry from a document, you might consider placing the document holder directly in front of your eyes and the monitor slightly to the side.

If you must perform other tasks in addition to using a computer, such as reading or handwriting reports, it may be difficult to keep your monitor and keyboard in front of your chest; they take up too much valuable desk space. Because it is not practical to move equipment around every time you change from one task to another, you might want to consider what is called an *articulating arm*. This piece of equipment holds your computer monitor in front of your eyes but allows you to swing it out of your way so that you can use the desk space directly in front of you. When you need the computer again, it's as simple as swinging the monitor back.

If you use a telephone frequently, especially if you use it while you continue to work with your computer, you may need to consider the use of a headset. This lightweight piece of equipment resembles a pair of headphones, with a small speaker for one ear and a microphone attachment. A headset is a much better option than holding the receiver between your head and shoulders—a position almost certain to cause neck stiffness and headaches. If you're on a tight budget, a less expensive option may be the use of a speaker phone if your office configuration and discussions allow it.

Now that you have positioned your computer and telephone close within your field of vision and reach, do not get too comfortable. You may still need to use other equipment in your office that requires you to move away from your desk. If you need to get a file out of a drawer, for example, use the wheels and swivel function on your chair to face the drawer, rather than twisting or reaching to get it. Better yet, stand up and walk over to it, because your back needs movement occasionally.

23

ALLOW THE HEALTH OF YOUR BACK TO SCHEDULE YOUR WORK ACTIVITIES.

Have you ever caught yourself putting off certain tasks at work such as photocopying, sending a fax, or even going to get coffee until you can do them all at once? Without movement, even the best chair cannot keep your back happy; your back hates to sit and not move. If you must stay seated, change positions as frequently as possible by making subtle adjustments in how your body is positioned in the seat.

An even better option is to stand up as frequently as you can to talk on the telephone, confer with an associate, or send that fax. Force yourself to perform activities that require walking around more often. Don't be too concerned with your loss of productive time. When your day is done, you will probably find that it was actually more productive than a day spent putting up with the aches and pains that sitting creates.

24

RELAX YOUR BACK.

After a long hard day at work, it is nice to come home and read the newspaper or watch some TV. You already know that relaxation is good for your back, but be careful that in an effort to relax, you do not put your spine right back into the same position it was in all day. If you work in the typical office environment, coming home and sitting on the couch or in the easy chair can have the same effect as a cast—holding your back in a fixed position and robbing your spine of its flexibility. What your back needs is a change in position. Read the newspaper or watch TV without sitting in your easy chair. Try lying down on your stomach, resting either on your elbows or on a small pillow to raise your upper body off of the floor. This position introduces the normal inward curve back into your low back, and you may be surprised how good it feels. If your job has you standing on your feet much of the day, then sitting is probably a good activity for your back, but be sure that you are sitting in the proper position (see remedy 8).

25

START EXERCISING REGULARLY BUT SENSIBLY.

There is nothing more important to the health of your back than exercise. Exercise strengthens and stretches muscles, lubricates facet joints, and feeds the disks. The appropriate exercise routine performed regularly and correctly is the best gift you can give your back.

Try to choose a variety of exercises that will condition different areas of your back and total body. If you have not exercised for a while, see your physician for a general checkup before starting your program. Also, if you are under the care of a physician or therapist for a concern related to your back or other joints, make sure they approve of your exercise regimen. Some exercises can increase your pain or make your situation worse, so let your health-care consultant guide you to the best ones for you.

As you start an exercise program, remember: You did not get out of shape in a day or a week; you will not get back into shape that quickly either. Therefore, start off slowly and be patient. Starting off too quickly will only increase soreness. To begin with, do your exercises three days per week, skipping a day between exercise days. As you progress, you can incorporate many of the specific exercises mentioned later into your daily routine without concern. Until your body is ready for that, just play it safe—pace yourself.

These exercises are not designed to make you a competitive athlete. They are intended to feed your spine and keep it healthy. If any of the exercises give you stabbing or sharp pain; cause any sensations like burning, tingling, or pins and needles; or cause any other abnormal sensation, stop the activity immediately and see your physician before continuing.

TAKE YOUR BACK FOR A WALK.

Walking may be the best activity for your spine and one of the easiest exercises to incorporate into your daily routine. The walking motion uses many of the muscles of the back, and as these muscles turn on and off, they gently pull and move the bones in your spine. These movements strengthen the muscles and lubricate the facet joints. Your walk should start slowly for about the first five minutes and then progress to a moderately brisk pace. When you walk, pretend that you are balancing a book on top of your head. This trick not only ensures good posture during the exercise but also trains the muscles of your spine and stomach to hold you in good posture throughout the day.

27

BUILD YOUR HEART, LUNGS, LEGS, AND BACK WITH STAIR CLIMBING.

As your conditioning improves, you can probably move on to a more advanced exercise–stair climbing. The benefits for your back are many, but stair climbing is strenuous to your total body; your heart, lungs, and legs all have to work hard with your back to perform this exercise. Before starting this one, make sure you really have the physical fitness level to tolerate it. Pushing yourself too quickly can lead to injury. When you use the stair climber, stand up as if you have a book on your head. Too many times you will see people slumped over forward as they perform this exercise. Although in certain instances there is a reason to perform the exercise that way, from your back's perspective, you should stand up straight.

CHOOSE CYCLING OR SWIMMING INSTEAD.

Almost as important as choosing an exercise that you need is choosing an exercise that you enjoy. After all, if you can't get yourself to do it, then it's not going to help you. Pick an exercise that you can look forward to doing regularly.

Riding a bicycle can be a good exercise for your body. It works the legs, the heart, the lungs, and, of course, the back. You do have to be careful about your posture with cycling, though. People tend to slump when riding, because they are tired and should rest, or because they are just not thinking. Be aware of your posture.

How the seat and handlebars are set can make a big difference in your back position. Stationary and mountain bikes are probably the best types for your back, because they sit you more upright than road and touring bikes do. The latter types usually have drop handlebars, which force you to bend over and round your back. Setting the handlebars up high enough to lean on without slumping over is best.

Set the seat height such that you bend slightly at the knee when the pedal is in the down position. If you raise the seat too high, you can make your back bend from side to side and rotate too much as your feet try to reach the pedals. This twisting can irritate your back. As you ride your bike, remember that you are doing it for your back and your good health, not for competition. Keep your gears set so that pedaling is easy. Your back will get a lot of exercise without a lot of irritation if you keep it in low gear.

Maybe cycling just isn't an option for you. Exercise in the water may be more your style, and it can feel great on your back. Water supports your body, and when the temperature is moderately warm, swimming warms muscles and opens blood vessels, relaxing your back. Also, the motion of swimming uses almost all of the muscles in and around your back and increases joint lubrication and overall flexibility.

Even if you are an out-of-shape novice for whom swimming seems too strenuous, you can learn to use the water to your advantage. If you are not a good swimmer, try using a flotation device so you can stay afloat without exhausting effort. For example, a wet vest allows you to walk or run in deep water without touching the bottom of the pool. You don't even have to know how to swim at all to wade through the shallow end of the pool and receive the benefits of the water's resistance and buoyancy.

You can also swim with a flotation device. For example, hold one between your thighs to keep your legs on top of the water with your upper body. You can also get hand paddles so that you can move through the water with less effort while still receiving the benefits for your back. Be aware that the water, even though it feels invigorating while you are in it, does provide a lot more resistance to the movement of your arms, legs, and body than you may be accustomed to. This can tire you out quickly and leave you fatigued for some time. Start out easy, and progress more slowly than you might with some other activity, such as walking.

29

STRETCH THE SMALL MUSCLES IN YOUR HIPS.

In addition to conditioning, a good exercise regimen must include flexibility. Keeping the muscles and other tissues around your spine limber is very important. The following stretching exercises involve the muscles and tissues around your spine and those around your pelvis and legs that indirectly affect your spine's flexibility. Remember the correct technique when performing any stretch: Stretch the tissues only to the point of mild tension, hold the stretch without bouncing for at least ten seconds, and then, let the muscle totally relax. To receive the maximum benefit from a stretch, repeat it at least three to five times. Remember also that your muscles tend to return to their shortened position after you stretch them. So stretch several times throughout the day.

The hip stretch is a good starting exercise. It stretches the muscles around the hips and buttocks and on the sides of your low back. Lie on your back with both legs outstretched. Grasp behind your left thigh, and gently pull your left leg, with the knee relaxed, toward your right shoulder until you feel a mild, comfortable stretch. Let your arms do the majority of the work, pulling the thigh toward the opposite shoulder. Your leg should be totally relaxed. Try to breathe comfortably; resist the tendency to hold your breath. At the end of the stretch, relax the muscles by allowing your left thigh to move back to the starting position on the floor. Perform the stretch the same way with the right leg. Alternate legs, and continue until each leg has been stretched at least three times.

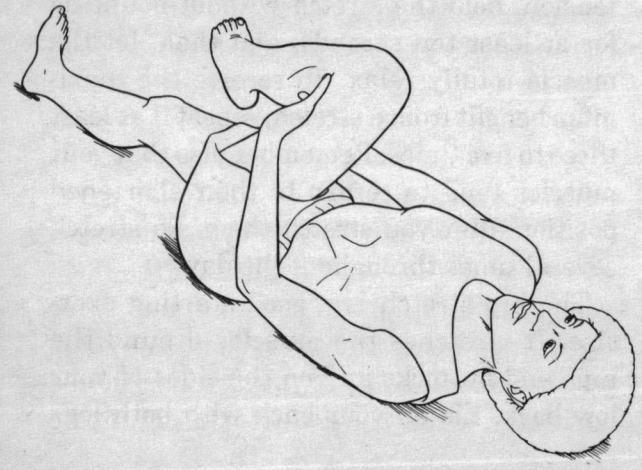

30

STRETCH YOUR HAMSTRING.

The hamstring stretch exercises the muscles on the back side of your thighs. The hamstring muscles affect your ability to bend forward; when tight, they can make it hard to tie your shoes or pick up objects off the ground. Tight hamstrings also increase the pressure on your low back when you bend. So when these muscles are not stretched out to adequate lengths, your back suffers the consequences. If you sit most of the day, this stretch is particularly important, because the hamstring muscles become shorter when they are kept in the contracted, seated position for long periods. By stretching these muscles daily, you will find that your back can perform a lot more work without as much discomfort.

Lie down on your back next to a doorway with your left leg outstretched on the floor, your right hip next to the doorjamb, your right knee bent, and your right leg going up the door facing. If you are positioned correctly, your right buttock should be touching the door facing. Keeping your right knee bent, place the heel of your right foot on the door facing. Gently press your right thigh toward the facing, straightening your right knee until you feel a mild stretch in the back of your right thigh. Hold this position for at least ten seconds. If you feel the stretch behind your knee rather than in your thigh, your calf muscles may be tight; they should be stretched before you continue to stretch your hamstring. Repeat the exercise with the left leg. Alternate legs and continue until each leg has been stretched three times.

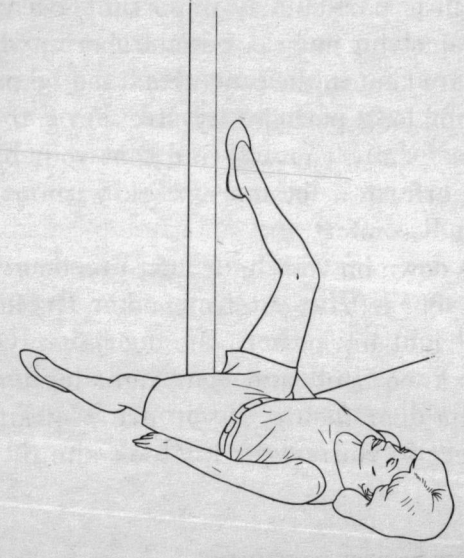

31

KEEP YOUR HIP FLEXORS FLEXIBLE.

You have probably never even heard of hip flexors, let alone know where they are, but this group of muscles is very important to the health of your back. The hip flexors are the muscles that work together to lift your thighs as you walk. When you pick up your leg to take a step, you are actually giving the signal to the hip flexors to contract—thus, pulling your thigh and picking up your leg.

What does this have to do with your back? When you sit a lot, these muscles, like your hamstring muscles, tend to shorten, and then when you stand, they tilt your pelvis forward. Your pelvis, in turn, pulls on your low back and drastically increases the amount of curve in your spine in much the same way that high-heeled shoes can (see remedy 17). This excessive curve forces the facet joints together, causing pain. If you keep your hip flexors stretched and limber, they will return to the proper length, and they won't tug on your low back.

To stretch the hip flexors, kneel down on your left knee. (Put your knee on a thick pillow so that it does not press too hard into the floor.) Put a chair or other support next to you for balance. Holding the support, put your right leg out in front of you so that your right knee is almost straight and your toes are pointed straight ahead. Keeping your upper body upright, gently allow your body weight to shift forward, bending your right knee, until you feel a mild stretch on the front part of your left hip. Hold this for at least ten seconds. Relax and repeat the stretch with the opposite leg and hip. Remember that you may want to do this stretch several times during the course of the day, because the hip flexors, like your other muscles, tend to return to their shortened position over time.

TRY A PRESS-UP.

Many activities reduce the amount of normal inward curve in your low back. This loss of inward curve may contribute to many back and spinal problems, especially bulging or herniated disks, and it can certainly be a major source of pain. You can help return the normal inward curve to your low back with this exercise.

Lie on your stomach with your body outstretched and your hands under your shoulders. Keeping your hips in contact with the floor, gently press your upper body off of the floor until you feel mild tension in your low back. Hold this position for at least ten seconds. At first, you may only be able to raise yourself a small distance off of the floor; don't think you have to straighten your elbows. In time, you may be able to press-up to that point, but take it slowly. It may take months to put back into your spine the curve that was lost over years. Remember to breathe normally and repeat the stretch three to five times.

ADD LUMBAR ROTATION TO YOUR STRETCHING ROUTINE.

Rotation is one of your spine's normal and vital motions. Any time you reach out with one arm, your spine rotates as your arm extends away from your body. An injury or a strain can, of course, limit your spine's ability to rotate, but some normal activities performed over and over to one side can have the same effect. Exercising your spine's ability to rotate in both directions will help your back stay mobile and pain free. The lumbar region of the spine is the part that runs through your low back, and its rotational flexibility is the focus of this exercise.

Lie on your back with your hips and knees bent. Your knees should be pointing straight up. Your feet should be flat on the floor with your heels up near your buttocks. Lay your arms out on both sides of your body, and gently allow your knees to drop toward the floor on the left side until you feel the stretch in your low back. Don't worry if your knees don't make it all the way to the floor before you feel the stretch. Only go to the point of mild tension, not beyond. Eventually, you may be able to go all the way, but don't push it. Hold the stretch for at least ten seconds. Then, return your knees slowly to the starting position, and repeat the stretch to the right side. Alternate and repeat the stretch three to five times on each side.

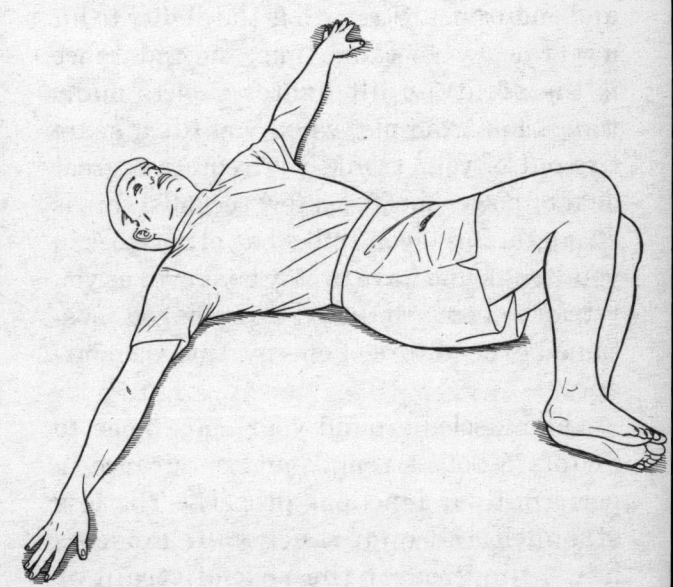

34

TRY A CURL-UP FOR YOUR STOMACH MUSCLES.

The muscles of your back support your upper-body weight, enable you to move, and protect the spinal structures from harm. While the muscles must maintain a certain degree of flexibility, they also need strength and endurance. Strength is the ability to lift a very heavy object one time, and endurance is the ability to lift lighter objects many times. For example, when you lift a spare tire out of your trunk, you require a great deal of power for just a few seconds; this is strength. But if you spill a bag of potatoes in your trunk and have to stay bent over as you retrieve them, you need a prolonged, sustained expenditure of energy; this is endurance.

The muscles around your spine need to maintain both strength and endurance to perform their functions properly. The less strength and endurance your muscles have, the greater the risk of strain or injury, and in the case of back muscles, this injury could involve the structures and tissues that the muscles support and protect—bones, joints, disks, and nerves. Keep your strength and endurance up so that you won't let your back down.

Your stomach muscles may be your back's best friend. They wrap three quarters of the way around your low back, and when combined with your back muscles, which complete the loop around your low back, they provide support to all sides of your spine like guy wires supporting a tower. If the wires on one side of the tower become loose, the tower will lean toward the wires that are still tight. This is essentially what happens to the spine when the stomach muscles lose their strength. Because they attach to both the ribs and the pelvis, when they weaken, they lengthen as the stomach is pulled down and out by gravity. This lengthening ultimately ends up causing a pot belly, or beer belly, appearance, and an exaggerated curve develops in the low back. The excess curve, in turn, compresses the facet joints, which scream with pain with even simple activities. You can maintain better posture, a better overall appearance, and a healthier back by strengthening your stomach muscles.

The best exercise that the beginner can do to strengthen stomach muscles is the curl-up. Lie on your back with your knees bent and your feet flat on the floor. Hold your hands together between your thighs and gently lift your head and upper body only until your shoulder blades are off of the ground. (A curl-up is not a sit-up, so don't bring your body all the way up.) Then, return to the starting position on the floor. Move slowly so your muscles get a good strength workout on the way up and on the way down. Taking it slowly also helps to prevent you from pulling anything. Start with 5 to 10 lifts, or repetitions, and over the course of a few weeks, try to progress to 25 to 30 repetitions without stopping. Use good technique, and don't forget to breathe normally.

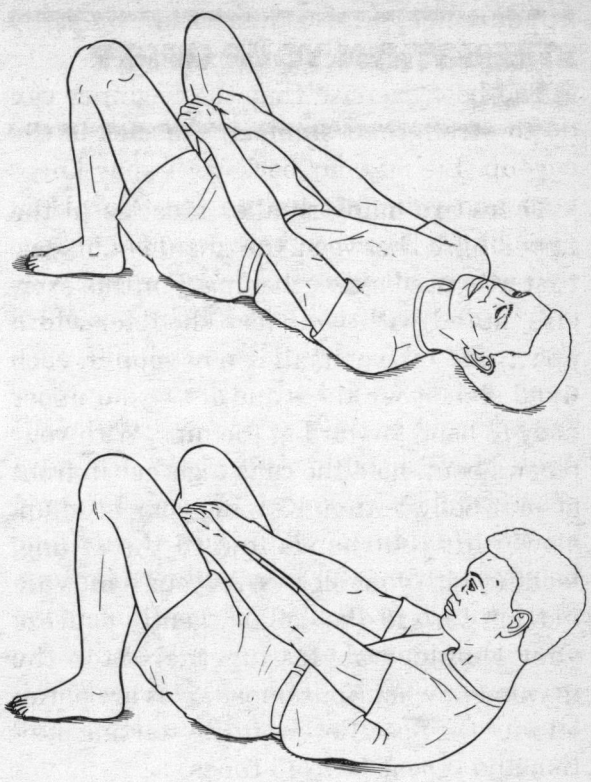

Lie on your back with your knees up and your hands together between your thighs *(top)*. Lift your upper body off the floor until your shoulder blades are no longer touching *(bottom)*. Slowly return to the starting position.

35

STRENGTHEN YOUR UPPER BACK.

There are many smaller muscles in the upper back, between the shoulder blades, that also need strengthening. For this exercise, stand with your feet shoulder-width apart and take a small can of soup in each hand. Bend your knees and allow your upper body to bend forward at the hips. With your elbows bent, hold the cans together in front of your belly button. Keeping your head up, slowly lift your hands toward the ceiling, leading with your elbows. As your hands are moving toward the ceiling, gently squeeze your shoulder blades together. Stop the movement when your upper arms are parallel with the floor. Return to the starting position and repeat 10 to 15 times.

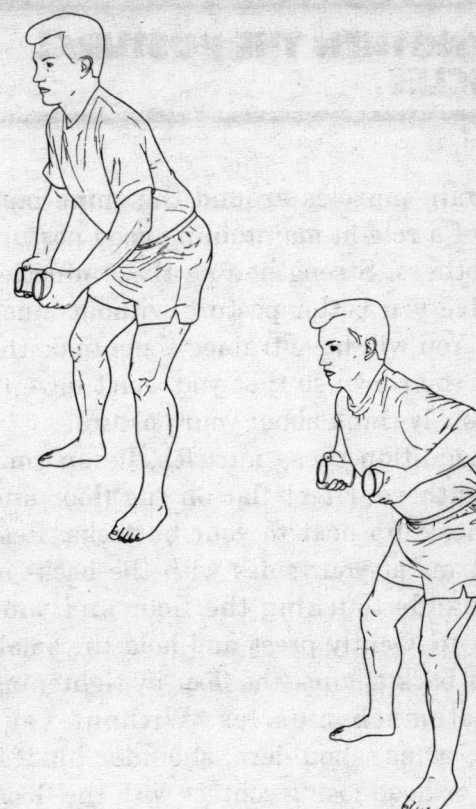

With your feet shoulder-width apart, knees bent slightly, and back straight, hold two soup cans together in front of your stomach *(top)*. Slowly lift them, leading with your elbows and squeezing your shoulder blades together, until your upper arms are parallel to the floor *(bottom)*.

36

STRENGTHEN THE POSTURAL MUSCLES.

Certain muscles around the spine play more of a role in maintaining good posture than others. Strengthening these muscles will give you better posture without much effort. You will have trained them to do the job on their own so that you won't have to consciously think about your posture.

To condition these muscles, lie on your back with your feet flat on the floor and your heels up next to your buttocks. Rest your arms at your sides with the backs of your hands touching the floor and your palms up. Gently press and hold the small of your back against the floor by tightening your stomach muscles. Without your hands, arms, shoulders, shoulder blades, spine, or head losing contact with the floor, slowly slide your hands and arms away from the sides of the body. Move your arms slowly so that you can monitor whether you are maintaining contact with the floor. Your goal is to get your hands and arms

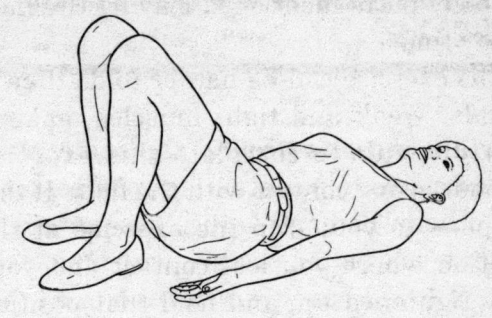

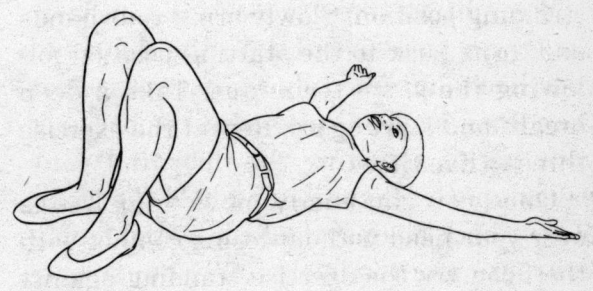

Lie on your back with you knees bent, your arms at your sides, and hands palm side up *(top)*. Without letting your hands, arms, shoulder blades, spine, or head lose contact with the floor, slide your arms up over your head *(bottom)*.

outstretched over your head without any of the body parts mentioned leaving the floor at any time.

This exercise can be harder to do than it sounds. Weak and tight muscles make it very difficult to complete this exercise without losing contact with the floor. If this happens to you, stop the exercise at the position where you lost contact and your body tightened up, and hold that position for about five seconds. Whatever you do, do not force your body into an awkward or straining position. Slowly bring your hands and arms back to the starting position following the same technique. Take a deep breath and start again. Repeat the exercise three to five times.

Once you can easily move your hands over your head without losing contact with the floor, try the exercise standing against a wall. Place your feet about six inches from the wall with your knees and hips only slightly bent. Follow the same technique, but this time, don't lose contact with the wall.

37

STRENGTHEN YOUR LOWER BACK MUSCLES.

Finally, it's time to strengthen the muscles that are mainly responsible for supporting your spine—your lower back muscles. These muscles are involved in sitting, standing, walking, pushing, pulling, lifting, and carrying; back muscles work all day. In fact, you really cannot move at all without using these muscles.

The strength exercise for your low back is much like the curl-up, only upside down. Lie down on your stomach with your arms at your sides and your forehead resting on the ground. Start with your head, and slowly lift your upper body off of the floor as far as you comfortably can without straining yourself. Then, slowly lower your chest back to the floor and repeat 5 to 10 times. As you progress, see if you can do 15 to 20 consecutive lifts using good technique. Remember to breathe normally.

38

LEARN TO SQUAT CORRECTLY USING THE ASSISTED SQUAT.

Many of the exercises already described prepare your body to perform more demanding exercises. Squatting is a demanding exercise, requiring many muscles to work together. Learning to squat correctly is very important, because you can use the squat technique to lift heavy objects without straining your back. The assisted squat will train your muscles to perform this maneuver correctly and build strength in some of the key muscle groups.

Straddle the threshold of a doorway with your feet slightly wider than shoulder-width apart and with your weight on the balls of your feet. Grasp the doorjamb with both hands at about chest level. Slowly lower your body toward the floor by bending your knees and hips and letting your buttocks stick out. Don't just let yourself drop toward the floor; go slowly to prevent injury and maximize the workout. When the tops of your thighs are parallel to the

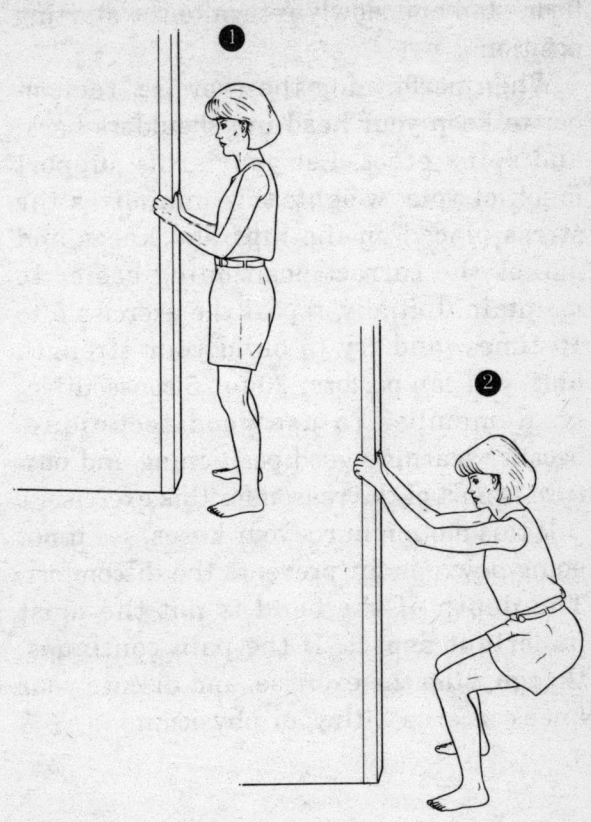

① Facing the door frame with your feet shoulder-width apart, grasp the frame with both hands. ② Keeping your back straight and holding most of your weight with your arms, drop slowly toward the floor by bending your knees until your thighs are parallel to the floor.

floor, stop and slowly return to the starting position.

When performing the exercise, remember to keep your head up, shoulders back, and spine erect. Let your arms support much of your weight; this minimizes the stress placed on the hips and knees and makes the correct positioning easier to maintain. Initially, repeat the exercise 5 to 10 times, and try to build your strength until you can perform 20 to 25 consecutively. Remember to use good technique, because learning good positioning and posture is part of the reason for this exercise.

If this motion hurts your knees, see if not going down as far prevents the discomfort. The depth of the bend is not the most important aspect. If the pain continues, though, stop the exercise, and discuss your knee concerns with your physician.

39

USE THE SQUAT LIFT.

No matter how hard you try, avoiding all the situations that may be stressful to your back is impossible. Sometimes you have to lift or carry things. Of course, as the weight of the object and the distance you have to carry it increase, so does the risk of injuring your back. However, the actual stress on your back is also related to the position of your body when you lift the object. Understanding how body positioning affects your activities is called *body mechanics*. You can decrease your chance of a back strain or injury by using good body mechanics.

Before you lift any object, you must first make sure that you are capable of lifting it. You can safely lift only a certain amount of weight. Even if you are extremely strong and you can lift 300 pounds by yourself, attempting to lift 310 pounds would be futile and hazardous—your chance of injury increases dramatically with every pound over your limit. So the first thing to do when lifting an unfamiliar object is to test its weight, or load. Pushing it with your foot is usually enough to give you an idea.

After you have determined that you can lift the object, position yourself over the object, with your feet about shoulder-width apart. Try to get the object between your legs, when possible, so that you don't have to reach out for it. Squat down, keeping your head up, shoulders back, and spine erect. The bending should come only from your hips, knees, and ankles. Next, get a good hold on the object, and finally, lift the object with your head up. Use your legs to lift. Your leg muscles are the biggest, strongest muscles in your body, and even though it takes more energy to use them, they can handle a lift better than your back can. Keep the object close to your body; lifting or holding an object up close to your stomach rather than at arm's length greatly reduces the stress on your back and spine. Remember that what goes up must come down, so set the object down using the same technique you used to lift it.

40

USE THE GOLFER'S LIFT FOR LIGHT OBJECTS.

Have you ever seen a professional golfer take the ball out of the hole after a putt? Chances are, he or she didn't squat down to pick up the ball. It would be a waste of energy and just plain ridiculous to use the squat lift for such a light object. Instead, golfers use the appropriately named *golfer's lift*. The golfer's lift is perfect for picking up small objects off the floor without expending too much energy or straining your back. With this method, all you need is some support (a chair, a desk, or a putter) to put your hand on to take the load off of your back as you bend over.

Here is how it works. First, face the object you are going to lift, and place all of your body weight on one leg. Place the opposite hand on a support, and bend straight over from the hip; your weighted knee can bend slightly, too. Keep your head up and your spine erect in a straight line. As you bend, let the leg with no weight on it come off of the ground in line with the upper body. This leg acts as a counterbalance to the weight of the upper body, making it easier to come back up without using the muscles of the lower back, which don't have the leverage.

You can use the golfer's lift for other common situations, besides lifting objects off of the floor. For example, you might be lifting a bag of groceries out of your car's trunk. Place a hand on the edge of the car, bend from the hip, grab the bag with the other hand, and lift. Again, if you let the leg without the weight come off the ground a little, you will notice how easy it is to get back upright. To make it even easier, pull the bag closer to the back of the car before lifting. Your back will not even know it's working.

41

LIFT MODERATELY HEAVY OBJECTS LIKE A CRANE.

Sometimes you are faced with lifting an object that is too heavy for the golfer's lift, and for some reason, you cannot use the squat lift. For example, you need to remove the dirty clothes from the hamper, but the hamper is too tall to squat over, and the one-handed golfer's lift just isn't going to do the trick; you are going to have to bend over to reach down into the hamper. Or let's say you have to get a large cooler out of the trunk of your car. Ideally, you would want to use the squat lift, but the cooler is at arm's length and down below the level of the bumper; again, you are going to have to bend. You can actually bend over with very little stress to your low back if you watch your technique.

The crane lift may feel a little awkward at first, but it is a good way to lift light to moderately heavy objects that you can't get any other way. Set your feet shoulder-width apart with your knees slightly bent, and position yourself as close to over the object as you can. Bend at the hips, keeping your head up and your back straight. You should feel as if you are sticking your buttocks out as you bend; this helps your spine to maintain the proper alignment. Next, grab the object and lift, keeping the object as close as you can to your stomach. Keep your head up and shoulders back as you lift. Remember to set the object back down using the same technique, and always concentrate on not twisting as you lift or lower.

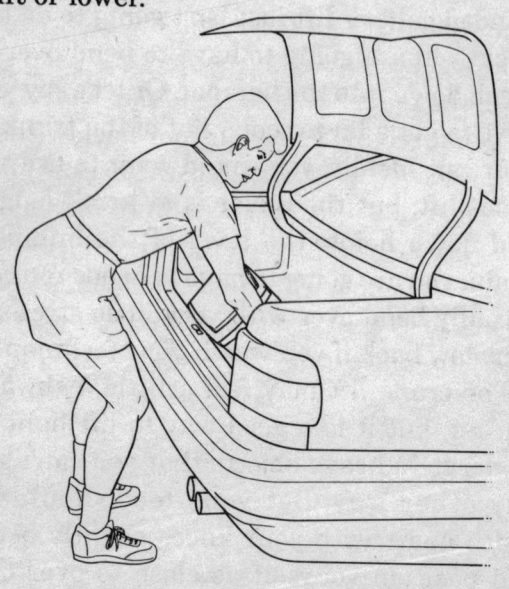

42

WHEN YOU HAVE A CHOICE, PUSH, DON'T PULL.

Moving heavy objects on a cart is, of course, much less strenuous than carrying them, but even with a cart, you can still hurt your back if you're not careful. As a rule, it is safer to push an object than pull it. When you push, you use the strength of your legs and your back to move the object; you can really get your weight behind it. When you pull, the tendency is to stand flat-footed and to yank, relying solely on your back without using the leg muscles. Also, the back is often in a poor position when pulling, increasing the risk of a strain. Next time you have a choice, remember to stand tall, lean into the object, use your legs and arms, keep your head up, and *push*.

43

MINIMIZE BENDING AND TWISTING MOVEMENTS.

The worst thing you can do to your back is to bend way over with your low back (at the waist rather than the hips) and then twist. However, many people use this foolish technique to lift and lower things every day; they clearly do not realize the long-term effect that this maneuver can have on their backs. Extreme bending and twisting are each hazardous by themselves, but not nearly as bad as combining the two motions. When you bend and twist at the same time, especially when lifting is involved, a large rotational, or shear, force is placed on the facet joints and disks, which dramatically increases the stress to these tissues.

Always try to face your work. This may sound obvious, but it can be very easy to sit or stand slightly to the side and turn just your neck or shoulders toward your work. If you have more than one piece of equipment around you, turn fully toward each one when you use it. Don't twist and reach for the screwdriver or the file folder; turn toward it and grasp it properly.

Also, when lifting things and carrying them a short distance, it is easy to forget proper technique and reach and twist instead. For example, a bucket brigade in which you are constantly twisting back and forth over a short distance with a heavy load is very dangerous. Take the time to take a few steps toward the spot you want to place the object. Use your feet to position yourself close to and facing the spot, rather than twisting and reaching toward it.

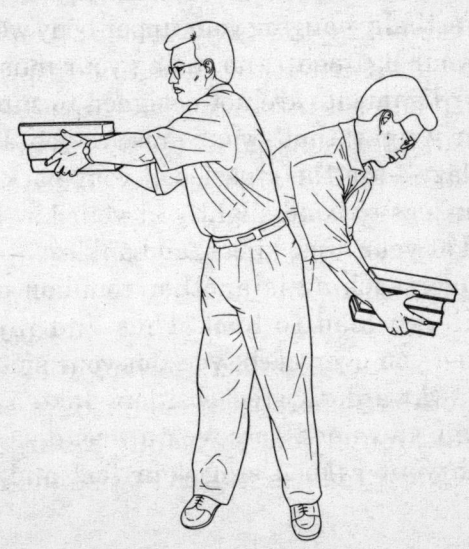

44

LET YOUR TOOLS DO THE WORK FOR YOU.

Tools are designed to help you perform tasks with greater ease. However, unless you put the proper effort into their correct use, tools don't yield their optimum benefit. In fact, using tools improperly can actually make work more strenuous for you and your back. For example, when you shovel or rake, do you stand straight-legged with your back rounded over the shovel or rake? If so, you are actually hanging your upper-body weight on your ligaments, not using your muscles. Your ligaments are not designed to support your weight; that's your muscles' job. Don't be lazy—use the muscles of your back and your legs to bend slightly at your low back and at your hips, knees, and ankles.

Overreaching is another common error that can lead to backaches and injury. When you overreach, you put your spine in an awkward, twisted position. Take a step when you need to cover a broader area with your rake. Using your feet and legs

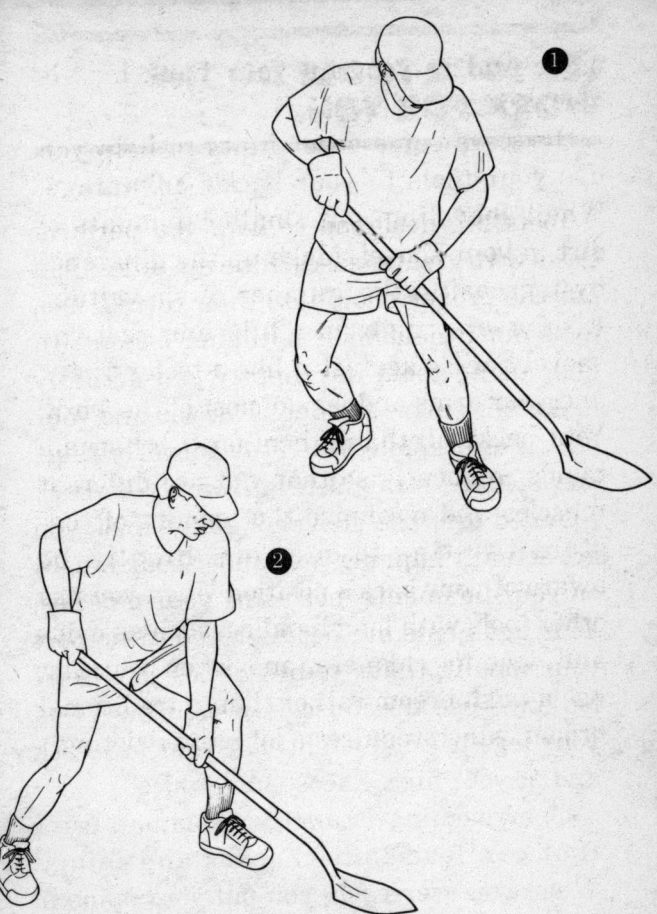

1 Using your knees as a fulcrum can give you some back-saving leverage. **2** Try to keep the majority of your bending confined to your hips, knees, and ankles.

more and relying on your back less is always a good idea.

Here are some other hints to help you use your tools to your back's advantage: When shoveling, put smaller amounts of dirt in your shovel. Make up the difference by increasing the number of shovelfuls. Also, use a thigh as a fulcrum; rest the shovel handle against it like a teeter-totter, and your arms and leg do most of the work. Your back will thank them for it. Alternate hands frequently so that you use different muscles and minimize the amount of constant twisting to one side. Finally, be aware of your back's position when you use other tools with long handles, such as mops and vacuum cleaners, and when you can, use a push broom rather than a traditional broom, which requires a lot more twisting.

45

PUT YOUR FOOT UP WHILE STANDING.

Standing for extended periods of time can be very stressful to your back, even if you do not have to lift, push, pull, or carry anything. In fact, it is the lack of movement in standing that usually causes low-back pain for many people. In addition to the inactivity taking its toll, gravity relentlessly pulls downward, stressing the structures of the spine. The upper body's own weight compresses the disks, pushing their fluid out over time. When the disks compress, they lose their height, the vertebrae push closer together, and the facet joints end up bearing much of the weight of the upper body. In the short term, this can cause pain, but in the long term, it can wear the facets out prematurely.

So much for the bad news. If you have to stand for long periods, there are steps you can take to help your back. The best thing to do is alternate sitting and standing if you can, but if you can't, the next best choice is resting your foot on a prop. Try placing one foot at a time up on a footstool or any four- to six-inch block or box. When your foot is elevated, the muscles of the front of your thigh and pelvis relax. Because these muscles affect the bones and disks of your low back, when they are allowed to relax, they stop pulling down and compressing your spine. Alternate feet every few minutes so that both sides of your back can rest. Your back will be better able to tolerate the effects of prolonged standing if you put a foot up. Now you know why saloons have a rail attached to the bottom of the bar.

46

STORE YOUR EQUIPMENT IN BACK-WISE LOCATIONS.

Sometimes we tend to conserve energy at our back's expense. We bend and twist just to avoid a few steps. One way you can reduce this tendency and give your back a break is to store things properly. Whether supplies and parts at work or products and tools at home, store things in places that are easily accessible.

Most of the time, people do not give any forethought to where they store heavy items. A heavy canister goes in the first open spot, even if retrieving it will require all manner of contortions. Or maybe that bag of charcoal just gets plopped on the floor because it's too heavy to carry any farther. Eventually, these items will have to be picked up again, and it would be a lot easier if they weren't on the floor or in the back of the closet.

Give some thought to where you store things. Place your heaviest items at waist height so you will not have to bend over when you return for them. Also, your most frequently used items should be placed at this level so that you don't have to reach all the time. That leaves lighter and infrequently used objects in the lower and higher locations on the shelves. If you have enough storage space, you could even leave the bottom-most shelves empty and never have to bend down to get something from them. With a little forethought, you can make it easy for yourself to use proper body mechanics in the future, possibly averting a strain or injury.

As with your most frequently used tools and supplies, set up your workbench, ironing board, and countertop at waist level when you can. If this is not possible, at least try to keep the surfaces you need to reach between knee and shoulder heights.

47

EAT POWER FOODS TO BOOST YOUR STRENGTH.

Most people see no relation between what they eat and their back's strength and health. Just like the engine in your car, your body needs fuel so that the muscles can continue to move and support the spine. If your car runs out of gas, the engine quits and the car cannot move. If you have not eaten, your back muscles may quit working for you; they can weaken, tighten up, and become more susceptible to fatigue-related injury.

Clearly, your muscles need food to maintain their vigor, but not just any food. The kind of food you eat matters. In our fast-paced society, eating right can be difficult. Fast food may satisfy your hunger and may even give you an energy boost, but your muscles and your body need power foods. Power foods are the ones that provide a great deal of energy slowly, over the course of a few hours. They can keep your muscles constantly supplied with the fuel they need to maintain the support and protection of your spine. Power foods are high in complex carbohydrates and low in simple sugars and fat and contain an adequate amount of protein.

Vitamins and minerals are also important; they play a critical role in your body's ability to release the energy from foods and in keeping your body healthy. Remember to get enough calcium and vitamin D to keep your bones strong and resilient.

Try to make fresh fruits and vegetables, whole-grain cereals, whole-wheat breads, and different forms of noodles and pasta the majority of your diet. Don't drown these foods in sauces, butter, dressing, or other forms of fat. Finally, limit soft drinks, candy bars, ice cream, cookies, and other sweets, because they provide too much energy too quickly for the body to use. Many times, this excess energy gets converted into fat and stored in your body in places you probably don't want it.

48

EAT REGULARLY TO MAINTAIN YOUR ENERGY.

Some people eat the right kinds of food, but they don't eat frequently enough to maintain their energy level and keep their back muscles working. The most important meal of the day is breakfast, because as you sleep, the energy stored in your liver is depleted by the brain and other organs. When you wake up, about 95 percent of this reserve is gone. Your muscles and the rest of your body are just about to run out of gas, and weakened muscles can quickly become injured muscles. So eat a good breakfast, and give your body and back energy they need for the morning.

Now that you've started the day with a full tank of gas, you must maintain your energy level throughout the day. The body actually works better and weight control is easier if you eat meals when you are hungry. You probably are conditioned to think that after breakfast, you should not eat until noon. However, your body may actually need the energy at 10 A.M.; if you wait until noon, you are starving your body for two hours and increasing the risk of a fatigue-related injury. This does not necessarily mean that you should eat constantly all day, nor does it mean that every time you are hungry you should sit down to a full meal. A slice of whole-wheat bread, a piece of fruit, or some low-fat yogurt may work just fine to keep your energy up and tide you over until you can have a complete meal.

Most people still believe in the three-meal diet, but a normal body should actually consume five or six small meals per day rather than two or three large ones. Research has shown that the routine of smaller, more frequent meals is much more effective in meeting the body's energy needs and reducing the storage of body fat than the traditional three-meal diet. Just be sure that you choose healthy foods for your six small meals.

RECOGNIZE WHEN YOUR MIND AND MUSCLES ARE STRESSED.

Lifting is not the only kind of stress that can hurt your back. Mental or emotional stress can be just as damaging, and many people encounter stressful situations daily. In the short term, the tension created by emotional stress can give you a backache; in the long term, it can set you up for a serious back injury, among other, more life-threatening health problems.

Many people hold emotional stress in their muscles, especially the muscles of the neck and shoulders. You might know this stress as a tension headache that starts in the back of your neck and moves up and down from there. A bad day at work or an upcoming job interview can bring on that creeping tightness.

What actually causes the pain? Well, normally, blood flows through the muscles of your neck and back with very little resistance. However, when you are emotionally stressed, certain muscles may tense up and squeeze these blood vessels. Like a garden hose with a kink in it, the flow of blood can get constricted or even cut off by these tense muscles. When your neck and back are not getting their proper blood supply, they let you know it with pain.

In addition to temporary discomfort, more serious consequences can result from this stress-related tension. Because blood carries the nutrients and oxygen that muscles need to function, a reduction in the blood flow can cause the muscles to weaken. They are, in effect, losing their fuel supply, and as mentioned previously, weak muscles are very susceptible to strain and injury. Learn to recognize when your mood and stress level are affecting your physical condition. When you feel tension, be prudent—don't decide to rearrange your furniture that day.

RESOLVE TO DEAL WITH YOUR STRESS.

After you recognize the emotional stress in your life, how can you deal with it? There are many ways. Try to identify the people and situations that tend to bother you. Maybe you can avoid some of them altogether—that would be the best medicine. In reality, though, some situations and people cannot be avoided, such as rush-hour traffic, deadlines at work, or an unyielding boss. Some anxiety is just part of everyday life.

The next best thing to total avoidance is learning to anticipate these situations ahead of time and making the conscious decision not to let them get to you. You might want to plan a way to make the situation easier on yourself. For example, if you must go to the grocery store at peak hours, accept the fact that there will be long checkout lines, and plan a diversion for yourself; bring a book to read. If you just can't stand battling rush-hour traffic, plan to work out at the gym for an hour after work. You avoid the traffic, relax your mind, and feed your back all at the same time.

You might want to try cutting down on some of the habits that can aggravate your already stressed out condition. Caffeine and nicotine can have the effect of creating a sense of anxiety even when you aren't anxious about anything. Cutting down your intake of stimulants may help reduce your stress level.

Of course, there is always the old stand-by method for melting away stress. Find a quiet place to get away; close your eyes; listen to some relaxing music; breathe slowly and deeply; and imagine yourself at the beach, with warm sand and a gentle breeze. Sounds nice, doesn't it?

Acute: lasting for only a short time, but being relatively severe; used as the opposite of chronic.

Bone: the rigid tissue that makes up the skeleton; its hardness comes from mineral deposits—mostly calcium phosphate.

Bulging disk: injury of the intervertebral disk in which the fluid center begins to break out through some of the fibrous layers holding it in. A bulging disk can precede a herniated disk.

Calcium: an essential mineral vital to the building of strong bones and teeth; found in dairy products and green leafy vegetables, citrus fruits, dried peas and beans, sardines, and shellfish.

Carbohydrate: any of various organic compounds found in food, including sugars and starches, that are the major supplier of energy in the diet. **Complex carbohydrates** are those found in grains and starchy foods, which provide long-lasting energy; as distinguished from sugars, which are simpler in structure and provide quick, temporary energy.

Cartilage: a fibrous connective tissue that is somewhat rigid, though not as hard as bone, and only slightly elastic.

Cervical spine: the section of the spine that consists of seven vertebrae, located in the neck.

Chronic: persisting for a long time; used as the opposite of acute.

Coccyx: the bone forming the bottom of the spinal column actually made up of four vertebrae fused together; also known as the tailbone.

Degenerative disk disease: a slow, progressive deterioration of the intervertebral disks in which the disks dry out and lose their elasticity over the course of many years.

Ergonomics: the study of the mechanics of the human body and the efficient use of human energy.

Facet joint: any of the surfaces on the extensions of a vertebra that make contact with the adjacent vertebrae.

Flexor: a kind of muscle responsible for bending or lifting a body part.

Hamstring: the group of three muscles at the back of the thigh that flex and rotate the leg.

Herniated disk: injury of the intervertebral disk in which the fluid center breaks out through the fibrous layers holding it in.

Intervertebral disk: any of the round, flattened structures in between the vertebrae of the spine made of tough fibrous rings with a fluid center.

Ligament: a slightly elastic, fibrous band of tissue that connects bones and cartilage, supporting them and holding them together in position.

Lumbar spine: the section of the spine that consists of five vertebrae and is located in the low back.

Muscle: the long, elastic tissue found all over the body that shortens, or contracts, to produce movement.

Nerve: the thin, cordlike structures that run throughout the body, along the spinal column, and into the brain. Nerves carry messages in the form of tiny electrical impulses from the brain to the body and back.

Nerve root: the part of the nervous system where individual nerves branch out from the spinal cord through spaces in the spinal column.

Orthopedics: the branch of medicine concerned with the skeleton, its related structures, and their proper functioning.

Osteoporosis: a disease in which the bones progressively lose their strength and density, becoming brittle and easily broken.

Pelvis: the region of the body above the legs and below the waist, especially the hip bone located there.

Phosphorus: an essential mineral vital to the building of strong bones and teeth; found in meat, poultry, fish, eggs, legumes (beans), milk products, and whole-grain bread and cereal.

Protein: an essential nutrient important for growth and repair, regulation of different bodily processes, and many other critical functions; chiefly found in meat, fish, poultry, eggs, dairy products, and beans.

Sacral spine: the section of the spine that consists of five vertebrae fused together and is located directly beneath the lumbar spine.

Sacrum: the name given to the triangular bone formed by the five fused vertebrae of the sacral spine.

Shear force: a force applied tangentially (sideways) to a structure; specifically, a force that would cause two objects, such as vertebrae, to slide in opposite but parallel directions.

Slipped disk: a misnomer for the condition known as a **herniated disk,** in which the fluid center of the intervertebral disk breaks out through the fibrous layers holding it in.

Spasm: the sudden, violent contraction of a muscle sometimes set off by an injury, often constricting blood flow, limiting movement, and causing pain.

Spinal column: the stack of 33 vertebrae that runs from the neck to the tailbone and that surrounds the spinal cord; commonly called the back bone.

Spinal cord: the column of nerves, beginning at the brain, that runs down through the vertical tunnel of the spinal column and carries signals between the body and the brain.

Thoracic spine: the section of the spine that consists of 12 vertebrae and is located in the upper back between the shoulder blades.

Vertebra: any of the 33 individual bones that form the spinal column, or backbone (plural, **vertebrae**).

INDEX

Page numbers in italic refer to illustrations on that page.